Your Body Is Not The Problem
Your mind is the reason you are not fit

Onyekachi Udeka

Memoir Maven Publishing
Philadelphia, PA

Foreword

There are a myriad of fitness professionals, scientists and religious scholars who attest to the power of our mind and how our thoughts allow us to reach our goals or not. Just like there's super food for the brain, heart, lungs etc., this book serves as super food for your spirit. Whether you're new to fitness or starting over due to illness, injury, or a lifestyle change, Udeka uses logic and inspiration to get you moving. With quotes and real-life stories from everyday people and fitness greats such as Arnold Schwarzenegger, there's no excuse not to get started.

Additionally, at the end of each chapter, questions are asked to help you overcome your own excuses for not working out. By the end of the book, you will have created custom-tailored affirmations to recite when needed. Achieving your fitness goal requires diligence and dedication in order to see it through. This book offers inspiration and a plan to help you do just that.

In Good Health,

Antico Dalton

Drafted by the Minnesota Vikings in 1999, Antico Dalton is a former NFL linebacker and defensive lineman. Upon retirement in 2007, he founded Pro Speed Sports and co-founded Linebacker Camps, the first linebacker training camp in the country. He resides in Charlotte, NC and serves as its Vice-President.

Table of Contents

Isaiah 40:31 - They that wait upon The Lord, shall renew their strength; They shall mount up with wings like eagles, They shall run and not be weary, They shall walk and not faint.

Introduction

Maybe you've always had the desire to exceed your imposed genetic or physical limits. Maybe you've tried being fit but quit along the way. Maybe you've tried diets but they only worked for some time. Maybe you blamed your body because you never thought you could be fit.

We often think that our body is the problem when it comes to fitness. This assumption gives much power to the body, when in reality, the body cannot make its own decisions. Except in the natural aging process, the decisions of the mind will always direct the actions of the body.

The purpose of this book is to describe how the mind keeps people from being fit and provide proven alternatives so you don't get stuck chasing solutions where problems do not exist.

Chapter 1

Believe – How the mind is the problem

The advice "believe in yourself" has to be the easiest advice ever given. So much so that it passes from person to person without hesitation. Yet, self belief is still one of the hardest concepts to practice and it may be because the **mind interprets it as another cliché.**

Aside from having the power to interpret or create meaning, **it is often ingrained in the mind not to believe in the unknown; to doubt things or events that do not seem normal**.

If a person's habit (which evolves from concepts and beliefs in the mind) creates any type of problems that do not seem normal, they quickly experience self-doubt which spurs this search for external solutions, rather than getting to know oneself. **The mind can cause a person to see problems and solutions as external so this person has no reason to blame themselves.** The motive for this comes from the best intentions and often prevents self-loathing, but how can you believe in yourself if you don't look within?

Self-Knowledge

Some of us tend to frame opinions of ourselves based on past achievements or current job status. In fitness, you hear people framing opinions of themselves by discussing their younger days and all the fit "things" they had done (Chris). But people are not their past since it's past already and you

are not your future since it's not yet here. **Although the mind encourages us to live in these glorious moments, relying on them causes us to doubt who we are in the present.**

You must realize that you are in the present and you can choose to be whatever you decide in that moment by looking within. Which is the essence of being human- an ever-evolving being.

One cannot become fit without looking within. Fitness is a journey that requires a conscious, present and intentional mind, for an individual to actually believe that they can push their body to its maximum potential.

Living in the present

If you choose to align your mind with who you are in the present, you would discover one of the messages in that advice: believe in yourself. You would discover that your mind holds the power to make your body fit, whenever you decide to follow the process.

William Ernest Henley wrote in his poem Invictus- "I am the master of my fate. I am the captain of my soul" to emphasize this message.

As a ruler over your mind, you are in charge of your thoughts. And your thoughts create your reality. It is through your strongest thoughts that your mind learns to believe that you can do anything. Without self-belief, you might find it difficult to achieve any goal, let alone a fitness goal.

The Reality

Recently, I was at park where what looked like a 9-year-old boy was riding a bicycle with training wheels. He rode his bicycle in circles while his dad watched to make sure he didn't fall. The boy made a few turns confidently and his dad decided to take the training wheels off. Once the training wheels came off, it seemed to me that the boy froze and was simply too scared to ride.

The boy pushed his feet to make the bicycle move, but he lacked the same courage to ride like he did earlier when the training wheels were on. His apprehension made it look as if without those training wheels, falling was inevitable.

This boy was at least 4 or 5 feet tall, "which is exceptionally tall for his age" and the bicycle was no more than 3 ft. so he would have been able to stand if the bicycle headed for a fall. Even with his dad watching, it seemed as if the boy didn't believe that he could ride without those training wheels. The boy was probably not **aware that he could consciously control his mind, through thoughts that reinforced his self-belief, so as to ride even with his fear of falling.**

Maybe the boy was too young to understand his inert power. But it surprised me when I, like many adults, sometimes deal with the same issue in fitness. It's as if we are not aware that we too can determine how the body acts by consciously controlling the mind.

It also explains why some individuals **don't think that they can exercise. Some resolve to live a sedentary lifestyle to the point that they stop believing that they are capable of doing any form of physical activity.**

This lack of self-belief, which lives in the mind, makes it difficult for people to get fit. How can someone get fit when they don't believe that they can make themselves follow through with their fitness goal? In fitness, like other aspects of life, belief is the foundation on which many goals are built. It inspires action and creativity even when the goal seems impossible.

See how Claude Bristol describes belief in his book, *The Magic of Believing:*

*"You have often heard it said that you can if you believe you can. An old Latin proverb says, "Believe that you have it, and you have it.**" Belief is the motivating force that enables you to achieve your goal.** If you are ill and embedded deeply within you is the **thought or belief** that you will recover, the odds are that you will; it's the belief or basic confidence within you that brings outward material results."*

The Solution

Fitness is result-oriented and the body usually serves as
evidence of how fit conscious a person's mind is. These
results are first created by thoughts in the mind, long before
they are manifested in the body. So for you to create the
fitness result you want, you will have to change the way
you think.

Now, you might find it difficult to create these results when
you've always heard negative things said about your body.
Many people have heard and eventually rehearsed those
negative statements in their minds so much that they
they've accepted it as their "fate" rather than believing in
their ability to change their own body.

For those dealing with this problem, just remember that you
have the solution within you. Always remind yourself that
your mind has the power to change your fate in the present
by thinking and believing that you can be fit.

As CT Fletcher said "never accept the limitations of someone else" or, in other words, limitations that others unconsciously placed on you.

Keller's Way

History is different today because Helen Keller did not accept the limitations placed upon her. Although she developed disabilities when the average "deaf and blind" girl had no hope of success, Keller managed to recreate her destiny by believing in herself. She had every reason to search for external solutions since her problems were beyond her control but instead she chose to find her solution within.

Keller writes in *The Story of My Life*, how her friends and family "doubted that" she "could be taught" and Keller would have agreed with their perception if she had never met Ann Sullivan – her teacher and one of the few people who believed in Keller's ability to learn.

Keller's encounter with Sullivan helped her succeed. It appeared that Keller's ability to learn helped her to believe in herself as someone capable of doing much more. She went on to become the first deaf and blind woman to graduate with a Bachelors of Arts.

In Clement Stone and Napoleon Hill's account of Keller, they discussed how she made more of her life despite her physical impediments.

"Surely if ever there was a person who might have been expected to complain of unhappiness, Helen Keller was that person. Deaf, mute, and blind, deprived of knowledge of normal communication with the persons who surrounded her, she had only her sense of touch to help her to reach out to others and to experience the happiness of loving and being loved.

But reach out she did, and through the aid of a devoted and brilliant teacher who in love reached out to Helen Keller, that deaf, mute, and blind little girl became a brilliant, joyful, happy woman.

Miss Keller once wrote: *"If those who seek happiness would stop one little minute and **think**, they would see that the delights they already experience are as countless as the grasses at their feet, or the dewdrops sparkling upon the morning flowers."*

Keller had to **"think" and believe in herself**, even when her environment suggested otherwise. She must have recognized that she had the power to think in the present and direct her efforts towards success. Her thinking led to her ability to believe, which helped her direct her body to perform the tasks needed to succeed.

Have you considered the people who believe in you? Have imagined what potential they see in you? It's sometimes hard to get the mind to think and believe in those tough moments. When you are at this point, it's often better to rely on the mental strength of other people who believe in you as Sullivan did for Keller. It doesn't matter if you have to borrow your belief in yourself from someone else. Their belief in you could be the solution you need to get started until you learn to believe in your own ability. That's why some people find it essential to join fitness groups or find coaches who will help them learn and embrace the strength within. So find someone who believes in you when you think that you might not be able to follow through. If not, the mind will enlarge your doubts, causing you to cling to negative beliefs that prevent you from being fit.

Once you find your rhythm, your positive thoughts and beliefs will always give you courage to plan, exercise, eat right, and achieve the results you want. The body will simply act according to your thoughts and the decisions made from its influence. It's your mind and the decisions you make that determine whether you follow the path to fitness.

Like Henley wrote, you "are the master" of your "fate." So learn to think, change, and take charge of your life in the present because your body is not the problem, it's your mind that needs a little push.

Personal Game Plan

Problem: Make a list of your doubts concerning your fitness goal.

1.

2.

3.

4.

5.

Solution: Create a reply for each doubtful thought so you can say it to yourself when that thought is trying to dampen your belief in yourself.

1.

2.

3.

4.

5.

Remember that doubts are just thoughts in the mind.
They are not facts.

Chapter 2

Hope – How the mind is the problem

Hope usually comes after self-belief is developed in fitness. Once you realize that your mind has the power to reach your fitness goal, a new sense of positive expectation is created.

This expectation could last for a while but when it fades away, it usually does so because of unfulfilled expectations. This happens because of the little amount of hope left in their mind to continue striving toward the goal. That's why people start on their fitness journey but eventually quit before reaching their goal. Hope is so essential that W. Clement Stone called it the "magic ingredient to motivating yourself and others."

People say it all the time: "I don't have the motivation to work out or to be fit." Not knowing that the mind, which is already lacking hope, internalizes this comment and replays it every time the thought of exercise comes up. Soon, the mind flushes out all hope of being fit, leaving only past glories of when they were fit.

As much as the body depends on hope to function, hope is not physical. It resides in the mind with doubt, fear and failure (Jakes) but somehow counters them when individuals demand it through their conscious thoughts. This is exactly why many physical actions flourish when people are hopeful.

But fear and doubt operate swiftly in the mind. In fitness, it could be the fear of disappointment usually experienced when people fail at their attempt to lose a certain amount of weight, fit into clothing, or accomplish a certain amount of reps or sets. This failure can slowly affect one's sense of expectation (your hopeful nature) and reinforce memories that are sometimes replayed in the mind when thinking of that particular fitness goal.

Fear and hope both exist as thoughts in the mind – that place where all good or bad thoughts flourish. For instance, a failed attempt to get in shape could demoralize a person to the point that they begin to expect failure in everything. Their mind replays the "failure tune" and their conversations reinforce it. Even their attitude will show that they do not expect to win in this area of their life.

Assuming one of those pictures of sadness is a failed attempt to lose weight, the person might find it difficult to try again. Especially if their mind keeps reminding them of the failed attempt. Anyone in this situation has the right to feel sad but those sad thoughts aid the feeling which overpowers any hopeful thoughts "to get in shape."

This cycle is so common and dated in human nature that the author of the book of Proverbs wrote in Chapter 13:12 - "Hope deferred makes the heart sick." Those words confirm the internal strength of hope and how it can manifest physically. So the process to reach your fitness goal involves the mind first, before the body.

Solution

When you start working toward your fitness goal with sincere belief in yourself, you will have to fill your mind with hope that you can get fit. Your fitness goal is centered on desire, continues with hard work, inspires faith and is sustained by hope. It will test your character throughout the entire process and challenge the way your mind works. Getting in shape is not just about training the body; it also requires that you train your mind. It's one of those processes where your result is a direct reflection of your determination and effort. Hope can sometimes be the foundation of determination. If you don't think hopeful thoughts for yourself, you might not be determined to keep working on your fitness goals after failed attempts. You might accept defeat and those failed attempts to get in shape become your reality. Soon you start making comments like "I can't get in shape or fitness is not for me."

Hope in organized sports- Physical exertion at its peak

"Hope is the magic ingredient in motivating yourself and others." - W. Clement Stone

Let's take LeBron James' career as an example. When he joined the NBA, James obviously believed that he would win championships.

He came close to winning during his first stint with the Cavaliers, but they lost to the Mavericks in the 2011 NBA Finals. You can imagine how painful this experience was for James and his team after working so hard to reach The Finals. Instead of considering this loss to be a failure or thinking that the championship was never meant for him, James relied on his positive expectation to win. This expectation drove his decision to join the Miami Heat. It's as if James used the loss of the 2011 NBA Finals to reinforce his sense of hope that he could still win a championship.

He went on to win the championship two consecutive times and moved back to Cleveland with this obsessive hope and determination, that he could win as a Cavalier. James told every player from fellow All-Stars Kyrie Irving and Kevin Love to the guys just hoping to make the team what was expected during the upcoming season. With their expectation aligned to a specific goal, the Cavaliers won the championship against one of the best teams in the league, the Golden State Warriors.

Solution

Hope and positive expectation are two faces of the same coin, so it brings you value no matter how you flip them. When you expect to succeed at fitness, your mind becomes an environment where hope thrives. It's the kind of hope that tends to carry you through moments of disappointment, especially when you find it difficult to carry on with a fitness routine that does not seem to work for you.

Hope is easy to overlook but it's really hopefully thoughts that help uplift the mind when your fitness goal seems out of reach. It fuels your expectation for yourself and helps you stay committed to your fitness goal, especially if your mind is not conditioned to expect success. When you are hopeful and committed, you can truly defy the toughest odds.

Hope shows that you have believe in yourself. It shows that you have faith in the process and that you are willing work for what you desire. Hope in fitness comes with the understanding that you recognize your failed attempts to get in shape. But even with those fearful thoughts of failure, your mind remains undaunted and hopeful that your hard work will help you reach your fitness goal.

Personal Game Plan

Problem: Make a list of your feelings toward your goal. What are those thoughts that make you feel like it's hopeless to pursue your fitness goal? Ex.: I am too old. I always give up.

1.

____

2.

____

3.

____

4.

____

5.

____

Solution: Create a reply for each hopeless thought so you can counter it with a positive statement that stirs up a feeling of hope.

1.

____

2.

____

3.

____

4.

____

5.

____

Chapter 3

Faith - How the mind is a problem

Faith comes naturally after you have learned to believe in yourself while hoping for better. In Hebrews 11:1, faith is said to be the "substance of things hoped for, and the evidence of things not seen." In other words, faith brings the hopeful thoughts of the mind into reality. That's if the mind is conditioned for success by sincere desire.

Consider the statement "I would like to get in shape." This statement is an expression of desire but also an opportunity to set a goal. It's easy to assume that the mind will automatically create the motivation to set or pursue this goal because the individual desires it. But the mind doesn't work that way. It's true that "thoughts of the mind can become things" but things don't magically happen because the mind wants them to happen.

Things happen in fitness because the mind consciously directs the body to work toward achieving this desire which sounds a lot like faith. The author of the book of James wrote in chapter 2 verse 17, that "faith without works is dead." So believing in yourself and having hope can only intensify the desire to get in shape. While working, faith brings the desire to fruition.

Even with the strength of the mind, your fitness goal still requires conscious control for these mental superpowers to make your desire into reality. It requires you to be in charge of your thoughts.

Solution

Faith in fitness can be broken down into three categories – Desire, Optimism and Visualization.

1st Stage of Faith - Desire

This is how Napoleon Hill describes desire in his book, *Think and Grow Rich*. Although Hill talks about it in terms of wealth, I believe that the same principle can be applied to everything the mind desires:

"One must realize that all who have accumulated great fortunes first did a certain amount of dreaming, hoping, wishing, **DESIRING and PLANNING** before they acquired money. You may as well know, right here, that you can never have riches in great quantities, UNLESS you can work yourself into a white heat **of DESIRE** for money, and **actually BELIEVE that** you can possess it.

We, who are in this race for wealth, should be encouraged to know that there is one quality that you need to win, and that is DEFINITENESS OF PURPOSE, the knowledge of what you want, and a burning DESIRE to possess it."

Wealth and fitness might seem unrelated, but when given a closer look, you'll realize that they both require that you have a "desire" and actually believe that you can possess it. Your mind has to be in a state of utmost belief in your hope for success and faith that your desire will come through.

More important than that is the definition of purpose, "the knowledge of what you want" which Hill calls the "quality that you need to win." This quality also comes with desire. In fitness, for example, you'll have to know "what you want" because knowing allows your mind to create a plan that correlates with your desire. When your mind is in tune with your desire, it will cause you to seek ideas that will help bring your desire into reality. Assuming your desire is to get fit and you really want to lose weight; embracing this combination can free your mind to consciously plan and work toward achieving this goal.

2nd Stage of Faith - Optimism

Let's also consider the second stage of faith in another context. Described by Jim Collins in his book, *Good to Great*, Collins writes about the Stockdale's principle from a conversation with General Stockdale himself. Stockdale was an American General captured during the Vietnam war. The conversation is broken into comments below in order to emphasize the importance of each statement. Stockdale: "I never doubted not only that I would get out, but also that I would prevail in the end and turn the experience into the defining event of my life, which, in retrospect, I would not trade."

Collins: I didn't say anything for many minutes, and we continued the slow walk toward the faculty club, Stockdale limping and arc-swinging his stiff leg that had never fully recovered from repeated torture. Finally, after about a hundred meters of silence, I asked, "Who didn't make it out?"

Stockdale: "Oh, that's easy...the optimists."

Collins: "The optimists? I don't understand," I said, now completely confused, given what he'd said a hundred meters earlier.

Stockdale: "The optimists. Oh, they were the ones who said, 'We're going to be out by Christmas.' And Christmas would come, and Christmas would go. Then they'd say, 'We're going to be out by Easter.' And Easter would come, and Easter would go. And then Thanksgiving, and then it would be Christmas again. And they died of a broken heart..."

"This is a very important lesson. **You must never confuse faith** that you will prevail in the end—which you can never afford to lose—with the **discipline** to confront the most brutal facts of your current reality, whatever they might be." (Stockdale)

The second stage of faith, as described in the Stockdale principle, **calls for faith and honesty**- being absolutely truthful with yourself. The brutal fact of the expression "I would like to get in shape," is that the person expressing this desire is probably not in the best physical shape by

---

their own personal description. And being optimistic for some miracle transformation in a few weeks will probably lead to disappointment, discouragement, giving up or a "broken heart" as Stockdale described.

While the statement expresses desire, the statement is passive and inactive, suggesting that the subject is acted upon by another agent or an unknown something. Although they are honest and recognize the need to get in shape, their statement infers this expectation that something other than themselves can magically help them achieve this desire to get in shape. The person making this statement is not a doer.

You can still have faith but you have to use it as a source of inspiration to work patiently toward your goal. Faith is therefore a mental tool that you can use along with your desire to get in shape.

Instead of saying "I Would like to get in shape" this person could say "I am going to get in shape." This statement carries faith and the determination that this individual has the power to bring desire into reality.

Believing and hoping with faith that you can get in shape is a thought process anyone can bring themselves to think. Although this thought process can be difficult sometimes, consciously thinking about it allows the mind to process your desire so you can to make reasonable exercise or diet plans to reach your goal.

Honesty gives you power and it eliminates blame. Even if being honest with yourself means admitting that you are completely out of shape and the "brutal facts" seem to say it **is impossible to change,** remember that your desire and belief in yourself can drive you to have the type of faith that will inspire you **to work toward your fitness goal.**

You might feel discouraged because of the facts but it's important to start just because this feeling makes you feel powerless again. Being depressed, feeling powerless and quitting because of the "brutal fact" will only leave you in a worse condition. But faith allows you to recognize that you can take charge of your life through conscious thought. The story of Morris Goodman is perfect example of an impossible case that was resolved through honesty and faith. According to the write up from the film, *Miracle Man,*

"Morris Goodman was a successful insurance salesman. So successful, he bought himself his own airplane. On March 10, 1981, during his first solo flight in his new craft, the engine stopped, and he crashed the plane, crushing his spine, leaving him unable to walk, talk, swallow, breathe or move any part of his body except for his eyes. His doctors *believed he would live a short, meaningless life, if he survived at all.*

Morris had different plans…

What Morris had was his mind, and his faith that one day he would walk out on his own two feet, and make a full recovery, no matter what his doctors told him. Using the same step-by-step, goal-oriented approach he took in his career, Morris began to calculate the steps he needed to make toward recovery. He set a goal to be home by Christmas of that same year. He succeeded before Thanksgiving, just eight months after the accident…"

Now one reason this principle might be difficult for most people is the idea of instant gratification. We want the result and we want it by a certain deadline. This can be great if it helps you intensify the effort you put toward achieving your goal, like Morris Goodman.

But Stockdale's concept of faith wasn't restrained by a deadline, which would have caused him to give up or die like "the optimists." Rather, his concept of faith was based on the belief that someday he'll reach his goal of getting out of prison regardless of how impossible his situation appeared to be. And it's also indicative of Morris' belief that he will someday walk.

I am very optimistic, but I think it's important to be honest or realistic when it comes to optimism in fitness. The truth is that lasting fitness goals take time and require a lot of patience.

Your fitness goal cannot be impossible if you have the type of faith that challenges your urge for instant gratification. It is reasonable to think that a few exercises or a new diet will change your body by the exact time you want. While this is possible, it might also cause you to give up on the process entirely if it doesn't work. And it's quite possible you would also give up what worked for one person didn't work for you. Because we humans are so unique, we can't put our faith in the results of someone else. A good example is the story of Marc Webster, who trained and ate like the Rock for 30 days.

Webster's decision to do the challenge wasn't based on a deadline but "a test of determination and discipline. I have no aspirations to look like The Rock," Webster wrote on his blog, "and one month isn't very long when it comes to the physical results of eating and training."

Webster clearly understood that following The Rock's routine would be an avenue for him to stay motivated so he wasn't too focused on instant gratification – making some miraculous change in 30 days, or trying to make his body look like The Rock's.

It's wise to understand your body and work with it as best as you can. You can model and apply someone else's methods but understand that fitness goals are not instant. The best approach is to use other people's methods initially but improve it constantly and ultimately make it your own. As Bruce Lee said, "absorb what is useful, discard what is useless and add what is specifically your own."

Fitness should be a lifelong commitment to learn, grow, and improve every day. When you truly think about fitness as a health benefit, you will understand the value of patience and adopting fitness as a lifestyle.

3rd Stage of Faith - Visualization

Back in college, the recreational center at the Stephen F. Austin State University had a slogan – "Recreate Yourself." This slogan was catchy but I always thought it was meant to remind students of their ability to literally recreate themselves in mind and body.

It's important to understand this concept because creation and faith always work together. Most things observed in our environment began as a thought visualized in the mind. As Claude Bristol wrote, "even the best ideas are created in thought form before it's made physical." So it shouldn't be rare to think that recreating oneself could start as a thought in the mind before it's manifested in the body.

In his book, *Magic of Believing*, Claude Bristol put it like this: "We hear much about various stages of meditation, levels of consciousness, thought creation, the strength of our faith-all of which deals with the intensity or degree of power we send forth. Creative force comes only when a thought is completely rounded out, when you "can "visualize the fulfilment of your ambition and see in your mind a picture of the object you desire."

Visualization requires that you have a mental picture of your fitness goal. It may be that your vision of yourself is you looking 50 lbs lighter. Regardless of the vision, visualizing this goal will help you act according to your desire.

You've seen or heard of kids that watch martial arts movies and act like their favorite characters in these movies. Some go as far as practicing martial art moves and coining nicknames for themselves. These kids are able to do so because the movie inspires them to create a visual representation of themselves as their favorite martial arts actress or actor.

The same rule applies in fitness. In Arnold Schwarzenegger's book, *The Modern Encyclopedia of Bodybuilding*, he talked about his childhood bodybuilding hero, Reg Park. Arnold described how he used to study photos of Reg Park because he had the type of Herculean physique that Arnold "wanted to emulate someday." Arnold also explained that, "the first step is to have a clear vision of where you want to go" and what you want to achieve." In order words, have a "definite purpose or know what you want" as Napoleon Hill wrote concerning desire.

"Where the mind goes, the body will follow" is a favorite saying of Arnold's. "If you want to be Mr. America or Ms. Universe, you must have a clear vision of yourself achieving these goals. When your vision is powerful enough, everything else falls into place: how you live your life, your workouts, which friends with whom you choose to hang out, how you eat, what you do for fun, etc. Vision is purpose and when your purpose is clear, so are your life choices." Arnold described it further in his quote- **"vision creates faith and faith creates willpower. With faith, there is no anxiety, no doubt–just absolute confidence."** Your body is the physical expression of your faith. When you can have enough faith to visualize the "fulfillment" of your fitness goal that aligns with your purpose, you'll find the inspiration to literally "recreate" yourself.

Remember that it's your faith that motivates you by "giving you the willpower" to exercise on the days you don't feel like it.

Stockdale and Schwarzenegger are both great examples of people who prevailed because of faith. Imagine what your life would be like if you modeled these principles of faith and worked to recreate yourself.

#FitFaith

When down and sore
My mind will hum.
A tune of faith,
A rhythm of Hope
This work ahead,
Bears huddles unknown
Still I'll push, for fitness, by Faith….

~ Udeka

Personal Game Plan

Problem: What have you been dishonest about? What are the
brutal facts of your reality. Ex: I eat more than I should.

1.

______

2.

______

3.

______

4.

______

5.

______

Solution: Provide a solution for each brutal fact listed above.

1.

______

2.

______

3.

______

4.

______

5.

______

Chapter 4

Work – How the mind is the problem and the solution

Earl Nightingale once said that "the mind was like a garden" – a fertile land where we could plant, create, grow, manage, replicate, accept or reject thoughts. These thoughts often determine how people act and action is the physical process of working toward your fitness goal. It could also mean acting according to the vision you have of yourself being fit.

Everything we do starts with an original thought except maybe the unconscious habits we've adopted over the years. Joyce Meyer says that thoughts also "prepare us for action**." So if you find it difficult to consciously manage the thoughts in your mind, you might find it difficult to think and act on your fitness goal.** If you wanted to do burpees for example, the thought of doing burpees would come from your mind before your body acts on it. The same applies to nutrition. If you want to eat right, you have to act on the thought. Acting on it could mean cooking something healthy, buying or ordering.

The conscious management of thought is not any different than driving a car. If you have a destination in mind, you simply think and direct your body to act on the thought by driving you to your destination. **Thoughts and the mind cannot be separated, just as the mind cannot be separated from the deliberate actions of the body. That's why the body is not the problem in fitness. The mind is the main reason people struggle to get fit.**

Solution

This is what James Allen's wrote about thoughts in his book, *As a Man Thinketh.*

"Good thoughts and actions can never produce bad results; bad thoughts and actions can never produce good results. This is but a saying that nothing can come from corn but corn, nothing from nettles but nettles. Men understand this law in the natural world, and work with it; but few understand it in the mental and moral world, and they, therefore, do not cooperate with it."

In a nutshell, you cannot think negative about your fitness goal and act out positive results or think about not being fit and act according to the vision of you being fit. "Nothing can come from corn but corn" as nothing can come from a fit mind but a fit body. Because your actions reflect your thoughts.

Action can be difficult because it requires some sort of physical activity - a bodily movement produced by skeletal muscles that requires the expenditure of energy and produces progressive health benefits." (Hoeger)

However, this book is not meant to teach you the science of physical activity. Its sole purpose is to help you recognize the power within your mind. It is this power of the mind through thoughts, that sets you on the path to pursue your fitness desire. This desire becomes the goal that can be achieved by acting out those thoughts. When you act on those thoughts in spite of your inclinations to avoid it, you learn that you can succeed even when the mind is resisting. These little victories from fitness can also become landmarks that help you believe in your ability to do other things.

Challenges to action

Expounding energy: There is a fair trade off in the description of physical activity- being that energy has to be "expended" for "progressive health benefits." In other words, you have to exercise to enjoy this continuous health benefit. People avoid exercising or "expending energy" **because they consider it to be strenuous.** And while it can be strenuous, it still beats the alternative – carrying an excess amount of unused energy that could potentially turn into excess weight.

A good majority of people can handle the weight that eventually comes with this unused energy and it works perfectly for them. However, others can't handle it and they become overweight and may even suffer from health issues as a consequence. This is not meant to scare you but to make you aware of your responsibility to yourself because you rely on your body to help you do almost everything. So you have to find a way to keep the body active by expending energy.

Finding time

Finding the time to work toward your fitness is goal is probably the hardest part of the process. **Between working**

full time, cooking, running errands and cleaning, there is barely any time left to rest, let alone workout. Yet the body doesn't care. It does not consider how busy you are when it permits muscle atrophy to kick in or when it starts putting you out of breath because of a few flight of stairs. It's almost as if your body expects you to put it ahead of all other priorities since you depend on it for almost everything. This means that you have to figure out a way to make time work for you.

How Arnold did it

When Arnold was still enlisted in the Army, his tight schedule made it almost impossible to find time for exercise. So Arnold had to figure out a creative way to fit fitness into his already demanding schedule. Surrounded by rules, time constraints and other barriers, Arnold developed a plan that would allow him hull weights in his military tank so he could exercise at any break during the day.

This might seem extreme for some people and I get it. But the key to Schwarzenegger's success wasn't his tendency to be extreme. I think Arnold's plan paid off because he didn't quit at the first sign of these challenges. Instead, he developed a plan that would allow him work toward his fitness goal.

Arnold planned with his vision and desire in mind. "Vision creates faith and faith creates willpower," Arnold said. "With faith there is no anxiety, no doubt - just absolute confidence." Arnold was able to do everything because he used the power in his conscious mind-from there he created the ideal time management plan and had the willpower to act on it physically.

Arnold's plan makes a point that work is not just physical. Many great athletes will tell you that 90% of work is actually mental, created through the thoughts and plans made in the conscious mind. Vision is an attribute of the conscious mind or its mental strength and your vision of your fit self can make the physical aspect of work a lot easier. It'll help you plan accordingly, so you can work toward the image that you see for yourself.

Weaver – Using mental strength to help the physical aspects of work

Successful people excel at applying their mental and physical strengths toward a goal. This ability comes naturally to them while others like myself have to work at it. But I have been fortunate enough to learn from great friends and mentors like Chris Weaver who uses this combination more efficiently than anyone I have ever met. When Chris and I were in college, our usual routine was simple: class, work and workout. While I would eat at any opportunity, Chris would sometimes go without food until dinner because of his busy schedule.

On this particular leg day, Chris skipped breakfast and ate a small lunch at probably 1 or 2 PM, but he still came to the recreation center at about 8 or 9 PM to squat. I remember him picking up the 405 lb. slightly bent bar and placing it on his shoulder with certainty. With ease, he completed 6, 7, 8, 9, 10, reps, slowing down on the 11th as if to remind himself that he could do anything he set his mind on. He went for the 12th rep and completed the set.

A few seconds later, Chris almost passed out. But it didn't matter because he had achieved his goal of 12 reps. The only thing that kept him from quitting after the 11th rep was his mental strength – his conscious mind urging his body to work for the goal.

When I recently asked what was going through his mind on that particular day, he smiled and said, "I had to finish it." I think Chris worked for the goal he wanted because he knew that his outcome would be guaranteed if he didn't quit. Chris's outcome was not just about the 12th rep. That 12th rep was a way for him to challenge himself mentally. It was as though he wanted to align his body and mind so they could work in harmony to achieve a goal.

I am not saying that you should push yourself like Chris does because it takes exceptional mental strength to disregard feeling ill, just to accomplish a workout goal. But his work ethic is important because he was able to do all of these as a student. Not a professional athlete, not a certified trainer. It almost makes you wonder what you can do when you apply your mental strength to the physical aspects of fitness.

You do not have to be professional at fitness, especially when it comes to your body. You just have to honest with yourself and align your goal with your desire. As long as you work on your body, you'll figure out when to push it and when not to. People in fitness always say "listen to your body" It might not scream at you but it will let your mind know how far it thinks you can go. Like Chris, you will be able to align your body and mind so they could work in harmony to achieve a goal.

Exercise has been proven to decrease depression and improve self esteem. By committing to regular exercise and making fitness a priority, your inner strength and body image are enhanced and this helps to boost your self esteem. But only when there are realistic, attainable goals.

Your body is the vessel that has allowed you accomplish everything that your mind has ever thought. You might be great at your job, career or school as a result of your brilliant mind but you still rely on your body to be in the best condition to act on the thoughts in your mind.

Jim Rohn once said that, "humans are the only species that could see a goal reached even before it's started." Your fitness goal lies within you and only you can see it, believe it, have faith in it. You are the only one who can work toward it with a well thought out plan. You are the only one

who can align your physical and mental strengths and
commit to achieving your goal.

Personal Game Plan

Problem: What are your reasons for not making time to exercise?

1.

2.

3.

4.

5.

Solution: Provide a solution for each excuse listed above.

1.

2.

3.

4.

5.

Chapter 5

Self-discipline – The Solution

The previous chapters emphasized the value of thought toward action and how the mind, through thoughts, determines how fit an individual can become if they work toward their fitness goal.

But fitness is progressive and in order to maintain this goal, you'll need to have the self-discipline to work toward it consistently. Anything done consistently can become a habit. It's this habit that ensures that you never stop working toward your goal.

Difficult and beneficial habits often start with self-discipline and I would go as far as to say that self-discipline can be a remedy to the problems of the mind. It's also a means to an end in fitness. Self-discipline gives individuals the ability to "train themselves so they can do something in a controlled and habitual way." Doing it in a "controlled and habitual way" is important in fitness because it literally help you exercise or eat better consistently. These two just happen to be the main attributes for lasting fitness results.

Belief, faith and hope are all important parts of any fitness journey but it is self-discipline that sustains the fitness habit you need for lasting results.

Habits

Charles Duhigg mentioned in his book, *The Power of Habits*, that belief "was the ingredient that made a reworked habit loop into a behavior." However, Duhigg concluded that "for a habit to stay changed, people must believe that change is possible."

When you choose to go beyond your goal to create lasting results, you will be attempting to change your habits which, hopefully, will grow into new behaviors. While it's important to believe that change is possible for you, you must also develop the self-discipline to work for your fitness goal until it becomes a habit. Self-discipline first starts as a thought in the mind and it could quickly become a decision. It's this decision that binds you to the commitment you've made to yourself.

Habits & Thoughts

James Allen best described the link between thought and habit in his book, *As a Man Thinketh*. Allen noted that, "men imagine that thought can be kept secret, but it cannot;

it rapidly crystallizes into habit, and habit solidifies into circumstance." He also explained that "a particular train of thought persisted on, be it good or bad, cannot fail to produce its results in the character and circumstances."

So if you are constantly thinking and are disciplined enough to act on your fitness goal, you'll surely "produce the result in character" and eventually make it habit.

Charles Dughigg explained, "when a habit emerges, the brain stops fully participating in decision making. It stops working so hard, or diverts focus to other task." Soon, the pattern will unfold automatically." Just imagine how good it'll feel when you don't not have to make yourself exercise. Or do those things that you need to do to create lasting results. Even when you can't make it to the gym, you might find yourself doing bodyweight workouts to pass time.

Dughigg's description of how habit patterns "unfold automatically" explains why it is easy for some people to exercise habitually. Their self-discipline (which started as a thought) in relation to exercise, has "crystalized into" a "habit" which now unfolds "automatically" to the point where they don't have to make themselves exercise. I also believe that they are able to do so because they've gotten their self-discipline to the point where they don't require a lot of motivation to act on their desire. "They are now self-motivated. According to Business Dictionary, self motivation is defined as having the ability to do what needs to be done, without influence from other people or situations. People with self motivation can find a reason and strength to complete a task, even when challenging, without giving up or needing another to encourage them."

Mind & body Transformation

"Be transformed by the renewing of your mind," is what Paul wrote in Romans 12:2. Tobin Crenshaw further says that "transformation begins in the mind" and it permeates to other areas of life. If you pay close attention to the stories of most fitness transformations, you'll notice that those individuals began their transformation in the mind before it manifested to the body.

The thoughts of your mind are the catalyst for change and when you align them with your new vision for yourself, your body becomes a vessel that acts according to your will. You can also refer to your Personal Game Plan until you're self motivated. This will guarantee your success in achieving your fitness goal.

Self Discipline

Discipline is the foundation for success.

It can pave the road to greatness,

Turning failure from pain to pride.

~ Udeka

Personal Game Plan

List all of your solutions below. Each morning, and when you feel unmotivated, read and recite until your motivation is restored.

1.

____

2.

____

3.

____

4.

____

5.

____

6.

____

7.

____

8.

____

9.

____

10.

____

Personal Game Plan (Cont'd)

List all of your solutions below. Each morning, and when you feel unmotivated, read and recite until your motivation is restored.

11.

12.

13.

14.

15.

16.

17.

18.

19.

20.

Mind & Body

The body is home to the mind.

It is the essential element that brings all creative energies into form.

While the mind plays host to thoughts, Both still reside in the body.

Knowing this turns the body into a temple - the source from which pure energy flows.

~Udeka

Bibliography

"The Miracle Man - Official Feature Film Site - Morris E. Goodman." The Miracle Man - Official Feature Film Site - Morris E. Goodman, miraclemanfilm.com/.

"Rock'ing For 30 Days." Rock'ing For 30 Days, rockingfor30days.com/.

Schwarzenegger, Arnold, et al. "The New Encyclopedia of Modern Bodybuilding." By Arnold Schwarzenegger, Print

Collins, Jim. "Good to Great: Why Some Companies Make the Leap...and Others Don't." Barnes & Noble, Print

Hill, Napoleon, and W. Clement Stone. Success through a Positive Mental Attitude. Ishi Press, 2013.

Allen, James, and William Walker. Atkinson. As a Man Thinketh. Waking Lion Press, 2008.

Bristol, Claude M. *Magic of Believing*. Pocket, 1969.

Duhigg, Charles. *The Power of Habit: Why We Do What We Do in Life and Business*. Random House, 2012.

Hill, Napoleon. *Think and Grow Rich*. Wilshire Book Company, 1966.

Hoeger, Werner W. K., and Sharon A. Hoeger. *Fitness and Wellness*. Thomson/Wadsworth, 2007.

Keep In Touch

If you were motivated by this book, please leave a review.

And be sure to keep in touch @onyekachi_udeka on Facebook and Twitter.

www.ingramcontent.com/pod-product-compliance
Lightning Source LLC
Chambersburg PA
CBHW060208260726
48658CB00005BA/1943